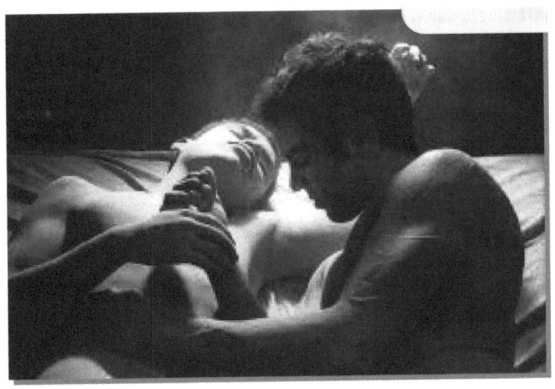

How to Share the Truth

A Compelling Look at how to share your
HIV status with your sexual partners

Written and Researched
by
Bradley Fowler, MA, MSc.

Talking About an HIV Status Is Not Easy

First Edition
ISBN 13: 978-1468008388

PRINTED IN
United States of America

Developed By

Construction EMarketing & Bradley Fowler, MA, MSc.

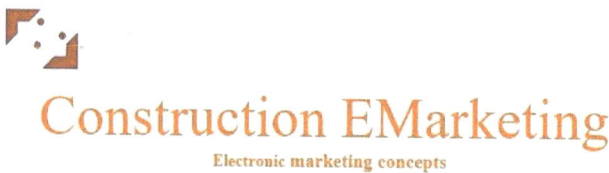

Construction EMarketing
Electronic marketing concepts

TABLE OF CONTENTS

Introduction

While reading a copy of POZ Magazine, the leading news source for the HIV community; I found myself engulfed with an article regarding the issue of disclosure and those infected with HIV, and the value of disclosing an HIV status to sexual partners. This thought-evoking article conveyed details about the continued enactment of judicial laws being passed and implemented around the world, in an effort to encourage HIV disclosure, with hopes that doing so will help combat the growing HIV infection rate. But what caught my attention the most, was the proposed idea that asking people to disclose their HIV status to potential sexual partners, could very well cause many people living with HIV grief; and in some instances, evoke many to continue remaining silent because they fear being rejected by someone, they like and/or admire.

I also found the statistics on the number of those being newly diagnosed with HIV around the globe interesting. As a result, I couldn't help pondering why people aren't taking more precaution about not only educating themselves on how to prevent being infected with the HIV virus, but also about abstaining from unprotected sex, and/or learning better methods to use condoms during sexual intercourse. Additionally, this article evoked me to recall how ashamed I was after I tested positive; and how ashamed I was to share my HIV status with others. Thus, to everyone living with HIV reading this book of inspiration; I assure you that I completely understand your discomfort when faced with the issue of disclosing your HIV status with sexual partners, especially if you were recently informed that you tested positive.

However, to help you combat that fear of disclosure, I think it's time everyone living with HIV, take a serious look at what we have been given, and our role in helping deter, if not, diminish the spread of the HIV virus worldwide. I also want to encourage everyone living with HIV to cease their fear and feelings of shame. After all, you were victimized by someone you trusted. Thus, don't carry shame of being positive; instead, let's fight to help protect others from walking a mile in our shoes and being victimized themselves.

In fact, it wasn't until after I completed the basic training course on HIV Education and Counseling, through the Michigan State Department of Community Health, did I begin building the tenacity to stand in front of a group of strangers and expose my truth…I'm HIV positive. Of course, before acquiring this knowledge and clarity about the HIV virus; I remember seeking every resource possible to better educate myself, in order to better educate others. Once I acquired the knowledge about HIV and how it is spread and how to prevent others from being infected by me, if we are sexual engaged. I felt compelled to share the most vital and intimate aspects of being HIV positive, with others. I thought doing so would be the best remedy to rid myself of fear.

Of course, it took years before I felt compelled to disclose my status with anyone, including family and close friends. However today, I no longer fear what others think about my HIV status, and neither should you fear what others think about yours. Of course, in some instances there are going to be people who will reject you after learning about your HIV status. But their fear of HIV derives from a lack of knowledge on the facts. This is why it's important, you take the initiative to stand up and speak out. Learning all you can to help others understand this virus, is the best method to educating our communities and those we are forced to share our status with. Otherwise, we are advocating for the continued spread of a virus that has no known cure.

As a result, within this book of inspiration are some valuable ideas to consider; and hopefully encourage you to rebuild self-courage, regain self-worth, and reignite your self-esteem, in order for you to relinquish your fear about disclosing your HIV status with others. I mean let's be honest, isn't it easier to accept your HIV status when someone else embraces you, despite you being infected? After all, when you think about it, even you were shocked when you learned you tested positive. So, imagine how others feel when they are presented with such information. It's funny though, personally, I thought being infected with this virus was going to be the worse thing to ever happen in my life.

But as time past and the reality of being infected set in, I learned that in order for me to regain happiness I had to completely embrace this virus. Of course, learning to embrace this virus wasn't easy. However, with persistence, you can certainly embrace the virus in you. The only thing you need to overcome is your fear of talking about your HIV status with sexual partners.

In fact, experience has proven that embracing the truth makes it easier for others to embrace you. And once you accept this basic truth, I assure you, learning to embrace everything else that comes with being HIV positive will be quite simple. Besides, once you reach your pinnacle of acceptance, you will have begun the process of rebuilding your courage. The key is learning how to let go of the past and taking the necessary steps towards building your future. This was one of the gifts I learned by becoming a trained HIV educator and counselor. Not only have I become empowered but doing so has helped me relinquish my fear of educating others about this virus. After all, the only way to help decrease the stigma associated with being HIV positive, is sharing our truth with others, intelligently.

Additionally, I felt compelled to compile some information on why disclosure may be the best alternative to decrease the global infection rate. After all, when those infected with HIV take a stand towards educating the community, it helps relinquish people's ignorance towards those living with HIV. More importantly, taking an active role towards helping others will prove to your community that despite our medical condition, people with HIV have a genuine concern about their fellow citizens; and most of us are willing to do what is required to help prevent others from walking a mile in our shoes.

Therefore, it's time you make a change. First, change is learning to stop punishing yourself. More importantly, stop punishing others. In addition, cease holding on to that fear preventing you from sharing your HIV status with your sexual partners. Trust me, once you reach this level of change you will become instrumental in saving the life of another.

Letting It All Go

It's funny, but during that very moment when you think you have everything under control, reality tends to slap you in the face and often sends you on a wild goose chase. Searching for the answers to overcome your pain. Yet reality seems to bewilder you and drive you further insane. And no matter what you do to camouflage your fear; quite often, you feel as though you don't posses the key ingredient to feel whole again.

But have no fear; no longer must you worry because the Universe is in control. This entity holds the power to relinquish the poison seemingly controlling your mind. The only think required is embracing your truth. After all, a portion of the Universe is buried deep inside of you.

Thus, to help you overcome the perils of life; through it all, don't ever forget the essence of love: the greatest gift to us all. The power it gives enables us the ability to let go of our pain and fear

and giving our worries over to a higher power: The
Master of fate, the beginning and our end. If only
for one second, please trust in these words my
beloved friends. God is the greatest, just believe and
have faith in HIM.

.

Dear Reader

Greetings! The purpose of writing this letter is to inform you that I'm living with HIV. Sadly, a few years ago, I tested positive. But today, I'm finally taking an active role in helping combat the spread of HIV, with hope of encouraging others living with HIV, to join me in this right-of-passage celebration.

Sadly, despite many efforts in the past to help slow down the spread of HIV; HIV prevention education has seemingly been ignored by many. After all, according to the Center of Disease Control-CDC, "in 2017, 38,739 people were diagnosed with HIV" (CDC, 2017). Seemingly, each year, more people are being infected with the HIV virus. In fact, worldwide, HIV infection rates continue climbing to staggering numbers. This proves that countless people living with HIV and are unaware of their positive status, are willfully, unknowingly engaging in unsafe sexual behavior that is increasing the spread of the HIV virus.

Moreover, this proves that many living with the HIV virus, knowingly are spreading the virus to their sexual partners, without disclosing.

According to the UNAIDS organization Website on July 7th, 2019, 36.9 million people are living with HIV worldwide since 2017 (UNAIDS, 2019). Sadly, before a cure can be found, don't you agree that it's imperative for those who are living with the HIV virus, to take the initiative to share their HIV status with sexual partners, in an effort to help stop the spread of this virus? If not, if laws have been enacted to evoke disclosure. What if laws were enacted to separate those living with HIV/AIDS from the rest of society?

These are the issues we face living with this virus. Our peers who lack clarity on this virus, could very well begin rallying for better ways to deter the continued spread of HIV in their communities. What if enough signatures were collected and submitted to Congress, asking to impose strict regulations on everyone current living with HIV/AIDS around the world? How would this impede upon our right to love and live out lives free from discrimination? These are the issues we must concern ourselves with.

Don't get me wrong, after testing positive the idea of sharing my diagnosis with others wasn't a thought at all. In fact, for years, I refused to acknowledge that I was positive, and tried living as if I wasn't infected at all. I laugh just thinking about how terrified I was. But in order to begin healing, I had to begin acknowledging this truth and learning how to embrace the new me. Trust me, I feel you carrying the burden of disclosure, especially when it impedes upon your right to life, liberty, and the pursuit of happiness, is scary. But as years passed, learning to talk openly with others about HIV and my own status, became easier. In fact, doing so helped boost my self-esteem and eliminate my depression. After all, depression has a way of impacting the lives of those living with HIV, after testing positive.

In fact, did you know that depression is the second leading cause of death amongst people living with HIV? Or, are you aware that people who test positive for the HIV virus, think about suicide at least once after testing positive? Just imagine how often the thought of having sex with someone without sharing a positive diagnosis, crosses the mind of many living with HIV.

Take for instance, imagine being at a local night club or bar, and glancing over at someone you find extremely attractive. Immediately, the individual approaches you, orders you a drink, and starts an enthralling conversation. Afterwards, the two of you exchange phone numbers and schedule to meet. Question is, will you be honest about being infected? Better yet, will he or she, if he or she is infected, be honest an disclose to you?

On many occasions, this has happened to countless people around the globe. So often, just this past weekend, two people met in a night club, bar, or mall, and didn't think about HIV. The only thought, he or she concentrated on, was the attraction for the other person. Sadly, today the growth and spread of the HIV virus has reached epic numbers. In fact, 19.6 million people were living with HIV in eastern and southern Africa, in 2017 (UNAIDS.org, 2019). "6.1 million (16%) in western and central Africa, 5.2 million (14%) in Asia and the Pacific, and 2.2 million (6%) in Western and Central Europe and North America" (UNAIDS.org, 2019).

Unfortunately, each and every person living with HIV, has the power to help end the spread of this virus. That's the issue with being infected with this virus. People think its okay to remain silent about having this virus. This is why people continue infecting others and/or moving from one person to the next, without ever disclosing. This is why I'm writing this letter in hopes of encouraging you to begin taking the initiative to share your HIV status with sexual partners. After all, doing so can help prevent someone else from experiencing the same challenges, you are facing.

Thus, please cease being afraid to tell the truth, and begin taking the initiative to stand up for others. In fact, educating others about living with HIV will help decrease the infection rate around the globe. Moreover, it will give someone else the courage to begin sharing their HIV status with sexual partners. Therefore, I ask each of you living with HIV, to be the voice that helps end the spread of HIV. Thank you!

Removing the Mask of Fear

Many months after testing positive, some men and women acquired the courage to open their mouth and allow the words to come out about being infected with HIV, during an intimate conversation with someone, they were interested in. But for some reason, as they began to share their personal testimony, they stopped. After all, fear prevented them from speaking the words. And even though, they eventually reached the pinnacle of self acceptance in order for them to share something so intimate. Deep inside their mind, there was still something begging them not to do it.

In fact, quite often many living with HIV find themselves thinking back and pondering about who could have given them this virus. However, it doesn't make a difference who infected you. What is important is finding solace within self and learning to accept what has happened. Moreover, taking the initiative to begin incorporating positive activities in your daily life, in order to help you move forward, is a step towards building a new you.

And even after years of living with the HIV virus, hopefully you will come to understand that the most important aspect of it all: no one can free your mind from the fear you feel about disclosing your diagnosis with others, but you. So instead of pointing the finger at others for what has happened, learn the importance of finding the right resolution to decrease your fears. As a result, you will be able to accept this mistake and begin allowing the world to see the imperfect person you are. And it is then when you will be able to shout from roof tops: I'M HIV POSITIVE!

Learning to remove the mask of fear and sharing these words with you makes a difference in both our lives, and the lives of countless people world-wide. After all, finally sharing your HIV diagnosis with others, will enable you to set yourself free from feelings of self-hatred. Trust me, I'm so sorry, you tested positive for the HIV virus. If I could remove it from your blood stream I would. But realistically, the only way to remove this virus, is remaining adherent to your regimen and taking the initiative to educate yourself and stay healthy.

Thus, please take a stand with me in encouraging someone else living with this virus, to educate another. Better yet, be responsible and disclose your status, so another person can avoid being told, they tested positive for the HIV virus.

Everything Is Going to Be Okay

Learning how to live with HIV is different for everyone living with this virus. After overcoming the initial shock of testing positive, you will slowly learn to not allow your diagnosis to control the way you live your life. Eventually, as time passes, you'll discover the importance of talking about your diagnosis with others. After all, doing so will give you the courage to begin encouraging others to talk about their diagnosis.

In fact, once you reach that pinnacle of acceptance, you will understand the glory of freedom and how important it is to live your life free of fear. Surprisingly, I initially thought sharing my HIV status with others, would be the worse thing to do. After all, I felt as though I was giving people ammunition to hurt me. But I was wrong. Actually, sharing my HIV status with others, has helped me regain the self empowerment, fear stole away.

Truthfully speaking, sharing an HIV status with others, helps you begin restoring your faith in the power of love. Not in an intimate sort of way, but an emotional expression of sincerity for human kind. Believe me, when you begin to experience how invigorating you can become by showing others how easy it is to share their HIV status with sexual partners; you'll be happy you took the initiative to speak out in this fight to educate the world about HIV.

Take for instance, the day you tested positive, which for many was probably the worse day of their life. Hearing the doctor inform, you that you had a foreign virus that requires daily medical treatment that must be taken for the rest of your life, was scary. But guess what, so is finding out your going to be fired from your job, when that is the only income you have to depend on.

Eventually, you learn how to get pass the initial shock. And as each day passes, things get much easier. Yes, it may seem as though it's easier said than done. But once you come to terms with reality, I guarantee, the benefits of letting go of those fears and insecurities holding you hostage, will uplift your spirits and renew your mind.

Therefore, today, I'm asking, you to take another step forward and lend a helping hand in showing someone else the importance of sharing their HIV diagnosis with sexual partners. After all, possessing these three keys of strengths: love, hope, and a passion to change the world; will empower you to overcome the darkness preventing you from believing in yourself. The important factor is accepting the truth: you are HIV positive.

Accepting this truth will help you live much longer than someone who refuses to embrace this truth altogether. More importantly, accepting this truth will give you the ability to implement effective strategies to better your circumstances. Surprisingly, what you'll come to understand about being HIV positive, is how valuable sharing your HIV status with others, really is. After all, understanding how to cope with being HIV positive, gives you the ability to avoid self-destructive behavior.

Sadly, this is why so many people living with HIV, today, continue infecting others. Somehow, they find it fulfilling to inflict their pain upon someone else. But instead of them inflicting pain on someone else, they're making their own situation worse.

This is why developing this effective resolution was important. Not only does it help you overcome your fears. It will encourage you to talk about your ups and downs with someone else, who perhaps will understand what you're going through. After all, when you're able to discuss being positive, openly and honestly with others, you can begin to relinquish your fear about living with the HIV virus.

In addition, it's important to understand that testing positive is not a curse from God; neither is it a punishment for not living your life in compliance with religious philosophy, as so many people have been taught to believe. HIV is a virus, and with proper medical treatment, you can eventually suppress this virus in your system. Luckily, today there are countless treatments available that continue proving to show exceptional rewards towards the longevity of life. In fact, today's medical treatments have allowed countless people living with HIV, to rebuild their lives and gain the self empowerment they need, to finally overcome the social stigmas often inflicted upon them because of their HIV status. Yet for many of those who haven't reached this level of renewal, continue to have patience and you, too, will eventually find solace. The key is ignoring the stigmas associated with being HIV positive.

Additionally, I cannot stress enough the importance of staying true to your self and ignoring all negative ideology, when it comes to living with HIV. After all, living with HIV is manageable; you just have to be willing to do your part. More importantly, you must be willing to begin learning how to accept you, in order for someone else to accept you. Once you do this, the rest becomes quite easy.

No More Right to Privacy

Interestingly, the issue of HIV disclosure is becoming more controversial. So much, it has already begun to darken the door steps of many governmental officials, who believe the best way to fight this epidemic, is by imposing strict regulations and criminal laws to prosecute anyone living with HIV, who refuses to share their status with their sexual partners. As a result, I'm asking, you to cease your fear and begin taking an initiative towards educating the community about HIV prevention, (e.g., value of wearing a condom and/or not being afraid to ask your sexual partner, if he or she is infected). As you become more involved, eventually, you will learn that no one really cares about you being HIV positive. After all, there are enough HIV online dating sites available so each of us living with this virus, can find someone to have a meaningful relationship with. Despite these efforts, neglecting to share your HIV status with potential sexual partners, may eventually erupt into a horrible situation; depending on the state or country, you live in.

In fact, in many states within the United States, some of the laws enacted are harsh. Some countries even have considered separating those with HIV/AIDS away from the rest of society, in an effort to save others from contracting the virus. This is a huge debate facing the HIV/AIDS community.

Therefore, I beg of you to, please be responsible and take a stand on behalf of all people living with HIV/AIDS globally. If not, the outcome could very well affect us all. Take for instance, in an article titled HIV Carries Face Microchip Implants in Indonesia's Papua Province, there is talk about implanting microchips beneath the skin of "sexually aggressive" patients, to track and punish anyone who is HIV positive and neglects to disclose (The Guardian, 2008). Such an idea sounds ludacris. But ethically speaking, in countries where education on HIV/AIDS is outdated and lacking clarity to educate everyone, regardless of race, religion, and/or sexual orientation. Ideas can quickly become reality and influence other nations and countries to impose similar laws and tactics.

As American citizens, such an idea would certainly face a tremendous uphill battle in Congress. However, with states having the authority to enact laws and pass Bills, without federal government approval. This concept of tracking can be imposed in states that have high religious following citizens, who hold legislative roles in state governments and great influence on the voters in those states. Thus, it's time we all wake up, and cease assuming the law is on our side. Yes, we are protected to some degree. But if the infection rate continues to soar, perhaps these concepts of implants and tracking devices may actually become our new reality.

Relinquishing Those Jitters

Recently there was an exciting interview in an HIV magazine. At first glance, I thought the individual sharing her diagnosis with the public was insane for doing so. After all, during the time of this publications release, I wasn't as open and fearless to disclose so publicly. Yet as I continued reading this touching story, I realized it was time I, too, learn to do the same.

After all, life is about making new friends and sharing disappointing times with others, so they can learn from our experiences, in order to begin seeing their own hidden strengths. Moreover, talking about this diagnosis will give people the chance to embrace the meaning of hope. Especially when so many people lack the concept of what hope is. Don't get me wrong, I'm not an expert of what hope is. I'm only walking miles in my own shoes. But hope has many meanings so countless people.

As someone living with HIV, neglecting to

offer hope to someone else, can stagnate another growth. Thus, please cease your fear and share your truth. Doing so will set you free and give you the boost you need to become a better you.

However, if you're one with long term jitters and haven't gained the empowerment to set your mind free from your insecurities about being HIV positive, do the world a favor, go look in the mirror. If you see more than yourself staring back at you, call the paramedics because you've gone absolutely crazy. Other wise, you are just as important as someone else. And the next person being victimized is just as valuable as you.

Besides, whether you realize it or not, there is still someone in the world waiting to love you. You just have to be willing to learn how to love yourself. Most importantly, learning everything you can about being infected with HIV, will give you the power to not only empower others, but help you build the strength, you need to fight your insecurities.

A New Breed

The other night while sitting up answering messages on HIV/AIDS Tribe.com message board, I was taken aback by some of the questions people were asking pertaining to why I felt I needed to write a book about disclosure. Honestly, over the years, I 've developed this concept for various reasons. First, to get rid of the anger and frustration, I've been carrying around for the past few years because someone neglected to inform me that he was infected. After all, living with HIV isn't always peaches and cream.

Secondly, I decided to write about disclosure to see how many people would badger me about taking the initiative to speak up and out about being HIV positive. But more importantly, I wrote this educational tool to educate you on the importance of relinquishing your guilt, fear, and insecurities about being infected with a virus some gave you.

Sadly, most of us forget, we were the victim.

Although, we knew the consequences of our actions; like many, we, too, gave in to our feelings of wantonness, desire, and needing to be loved. As a result, we were manipulated into becoming a part of a new breed, which now is considered abnormal by many.

Nevertheless, in many instances, we are quite lucky. After all, we know our diagnosis and can implement special regimes to help us live longer. Sadly, many others will not take the initiative to speak up or even be tested.

Luckily, you now have the ability to continue living and striving to become better at this thing called life. Once you embrace this treasure, you can finally become the master of your own destiny. And no longer be enslaved by those who seek to infect your mind with negativity, merely because they don't posses the inner strength you have found, which is one of the most important aspects required to defeat living with this virus.

Meanwhile, despite being a part of this new breed, you also can continue living and soaring towards your pinnacle of fulfillment, without fear and without willfully infecting others. Therefore, cease your doubt about sharing this truth. Besides, you've already conquered the worse. Everything else from this point is all up hill.

Rest assure, within the body of this text is an abundance of joy to encourage you to become a better you. Most of all, you will begin walking in the richness of being a positive asset to your community. Trust me, being a positive influence on the lives of others can help you tremendously in the long run. So, I guess you can say, "You're blessed."

Blessed because, despite what you think, there is always someone else who lacks the strength and wisdom, you already have. And when all else fails, believe in what you attain from reading this book, because nothing shared with you is senseless or even useless, especially if you put the knowledge to good use.

Surveillance

A few nights ago, while visiting a very good friend; I noticed an old issue of POZ magazine on his dresser. Immediately, I was drawn to the blurb on the cover and picked it up and began scanning through the pages. While reading, I found an article suggesting the future of HIV disclosure, could very well include intense surveillance tactics. But not the average every day police surveillance activities though. No, this article mentioned medical implants that would track each and every move a person living with HIV makes.

Of course, I was quite disturbed by what I was reading. So much, the article caused me to evaluate the idea more thoroughly. And as sci-fi as it sounds, I couldn't help but think of the invasion of privacy this impedes upon. Not only will implementing such an unusual contraption seem absurd, it would be criminal.

However, with the increased rate of wild-type viruses rooting around the globe, and unseemingly infection rates, such tactics just may tame this ugly beast. The only problem would be getting those infected to volunteer for the surveillance device to be injected into their body. But then again, it might not be as difficult as we think. After all, once our names are cataloged in the system, our contact information is stored in a data base, that can help law enforcement locate you, pick you up, and deliver you to the location where the implants are forced under our skin. If this were law, how would we combat being victimized? Who would care enough to stand up against this threat?

And although, there have already been many cases fought in both criminal and civil court surrounding the lack of HIV disclosure; in many instances, most of those cases have not been successful in prosecution. However, if I wanted to report someone for infecting me, I would first need to prove who it was that did so. And if I've had sex with more than one person within a year of time, I would have to assume each of those I was sexually involved with was the source of my infection.

Next, I would have to request a genotype test be done on every person I'm accusing. However, if the courts do not make it mandatory for those individuals to submit to the test, there would be no other way to prove any of those I'm claiming infected me, were the source. After all, a genotype only determines the strain of the virus.

Thus, imposing any level of sanction upon those living with HIV for not disclosing their status; seemingly, was initially enacted to help decrease the spread of HIV. Mind you, this conversation began in 2011. It's 2019, and 39,000 people tested positive in 2017 in the United States. If you think about it, not everyone living with HIV has been tested. And in most cases, many living with HIV never will be tested.

Yet for the million who do know their infected yet refuse to get tested because they fear rejection from both present and future sexual partners; those are the culprits continually infecting others without informing them of their HIV status. Unfortunately, when you think about it, in the long run, this entire dilemma is upsetting. Just think about how many people are having sex around the globe. Now imagine how many are having unprotected sex. Now count how many people travel from country to country. Surely the statistics compiled during medical research studies are not always true.

However, if your government considers imposing strategically designed surveillance tactics, such as placing tracking devices under the skin of those living with HIV, this may very well mark the next level of truth in historical doctrine. After all, since the beginning of time, humans have used their power to control the masses in every way conceivable. In fact, slavery was imposed because countless people were embodied by fear and lacked the courage to stand up and speak out against such inhumane atrocity. Therefore, when you begin oppressing the lives of those infected with HIV based on a theory of belief, that doing so is protecting the lives of those not infected, isn't that defying the law itself…proven guilty until found guilty?

Yes, many living with HIV continue having unprotected sex without disclosing their status; how else is the infection rate still climbing? After all, the only way to become infected is to have sex with someone that is. So, despite what society says about surveillance tactics, this idea just might be fathomable. However, have you given thought to the idea that those living with HIV, are already being surveillance?

This is why I come to warn you. Warn you to be safe with your sexual excursions and to cease your ignorance about disclosure. If you fear disclosing your status with potential sexual partners, there are countless ways to gain effective skills to help you do so; just make sure you invest enough time and energy to learn them. Then, you won't have to worry about anything else.

In the Public's Eye

The topic of disclosure isn't new. In fact, this topic has been main stream since 2009. To those who have taken a step forward and disclosed their HIV status with family, friends, and sexual partners, I applaud your efforts and tenacity to put an end to the vicious cycle of ignorance encompassing the existence of HIV. I also thank everyone living with HIV/AIDS who has been in the public's eye and put an end to stigmas associated with being HIV positive.

Some years ago, I stepped forward and shared my status in a featured article on the pages of HIV Plus Magazine. Initially, I was terrified that it would haunt me. So much, I didn't rush to tell everyone that I'd been interviewed. But as the day neared for the release of the edition I was being featured in, drew close, I quickly learned that speaking this truth is a gateway to self-empowerment.

Finally, when the digital version was available, I clicked the link and stared at my photo before reading what had been published. Proud of my truth, I copied the domain link and posted it on Facebook, sharing it with more than 360 friends. Of course, many of those are personal associates from high school and friends of friends, I've met. But sharing this link with people in general was a key awakening to setting me free from the bondage being HIV positive places on you.

Okay, now that I've aired my dirty laundry for the whole world to read, will that change the way I'm viewed in my community, as a man living with HIV? Will my neighbors respect me any more or any less because I exposed this secret? Better yet, will people forgive those who continue having unprotected sex with perfect strangers, they met just days after testing positive, without sharing their diagnosis?

Surprisingly, there are countless people doing just that: having sex with others after testing positive, without sharing their diagnosis. As a result, the infection rate continues to soar. So today, I'm declaring that this epidemic stops with me.

In fact, I'm glad I've finally manned up and told the truth. Even though doing so may not get me a Pulitzer Prize or even a Purple Heart. It does give me inner peace. Fact is, I no longer have to carry the burden of sharing my diagnosis with others. If the world doesn't know that I'm living with HIV by now, it soon will.

Thus, my question to the rest of you living with HIV, refusing to share your diagnosis with the world: why aren't you sharing your truth? What are you afraid of? Despite what you think, sharing your diagnosis is a blessing. Not only will it touch countless lives, it will change yours.

Why Not Tell the World

Taking the initiative to launch a global mission to encourage those living with HIV, to begin sharing their diagnosis, may seem pretty far-fetch to some of you. After all, suggesting someone share their status with others, requires you to expose your darkest secret. However, doing so will help countless souls unblock that needed thrust of energy we require to help us spearhead towards a pinnacle of rejuvenation. Besides, no one enjoys being mentally and emotionally boggled down by negative thoughts and/ or feelings.

Yes, I understand that for some, after testing positive, you are reluctant to share your diagnosis with others. Even to the point, you don't mind keeping this truth hidden countless years later after the fact. Instead, you rather continue intermingling and uncaringly expose others to this seemingly incurable virus. At least, until your conscious steps in and begins to eat at you for being so hateful.

However, for me it was different. Finally, after letting go of my anger for being infected, I couldn't help thinking about encouraging others about how relieved I felt when I began sharing my diagnosis with others. Honestly, it was rewarding. So much, I'm willing to stand on top of the highest building with a banner that reads: I'm HIV POSITIVE.

After all, the duty of protecting society from becoming infected with HIV falls into the hands of everyday people, who often don't understand what it's like being infected. Even scarier, those everyday people are not going to be compassionate when they discover, you were one of those individuals who had an opportunity to share your truth but neglected to do so; for whatever reason you profess. However, it doesn't have to be like this.

In fact, no one should have to rally for HIV disclosure laws to be enforced, because those living with HIV should take the initiative to stop the spread of this virus, themselves. On the other hand, if someone is not infected, of course, they do not know the pain we suffer on a daily basis, mentally and emotionally. And truthfully speaking, in many instances, most people could careless how we feel, because to them, we are monsters walking amongst the living with a virus that has the power to kill.

Still, that's not a good enough reason to continue infecting others. In fact, for those of you who willingly are infecting someone else without sharing your diagnosis, your actions are falling back on everyone else living with HIV. So please, stop being selfish! Be the woman or man, you are and stop waddling in self-pity.

If you need to talk about being positive, log on to Poz.com or hivpassion.net, and find a mentor or new chat buddy. But please, cease your ignorance. You and I have been blessed with the gift of modern medicine to help us combat this hideous virus. So, why continue taking that for granted? What happens when the funding dries up and the pills no longer are effective…something we all need to think about.

It's Not the End of Your World

Testing HIV positive is not the end of the world. In fact, it's merely the beginning of a new world for you. No longer will there be a need to invest your precious energy in what's wrong with your life. Better yet, no longer should there be a need to carry the world's problems around on your shoulders. After all, you didn't create them.

Therefore, today, it's time you begin rejuvenating and redirecting your path. As a matter of fact, it's time you begin taking pleasure in everything you see and do. But first, you must relinquish any hate you have that's keeping you stagnated. In fact, now is the time for you to begin living!

Ideally, in order for you to begin living, you need instructions. Not some step-by-step instructions put together in a scheme to entice you to purchase a book. But a compassionate and easy to relate to guide that offers substance that instantly motivates you. Yes, it's time you envelope the energy pouring from the pages of this book and become inspired to share your HIV diagnosis with others.

After all, doing so will finally free you from that mental state of "self-dislike", and help you escape the negativity clouding your mind trying to make you give up hope. Not only will you become inspired to finally tell the world, your HIV positive, by the time you finish reading this book. But, you'll finally begin realizing just how trivial you've been about sharing your HIV diagnosis with others. Besides, living with HIV is simple, you just do it. Therefore, stop badgering yourself about why it had to happen to you, it did; get over it.

As the days go by, please be sure to take your medicine if its been prescribed. Additionally, do some exercise at least three days a week, and by all means, eat right: veggies, vitamins, and clean meats. Furthermore, please continue to have good sex. But remember, you must tell everyone your lying down with, you are HIV positive. And don't forget-wear condoms. In fact, I found some non-

latex condoms at Walmart, that offers sensitivity
unlike any condom I've ever used. And believe me,
I'm not much into wearing condoms. But if it's
required to get to those cookies, trust me, put it on.

Let's Talk About HIV Disclosure

Talking about HIV disclosure is a difficult subject matter for many people, even those who aren't living with the virus. To some, its taboo; you just don't bring it up. To others, it's a topic worth discussing. But just sitting around the table dishing tea about living with HIV/AIDS can be upsetting. In fact, I recall a friendly get together I attended last summer over a good buddy of mine. He, too, is HIV positive, and everyone else that was sitting at the table I sat at is HIV positive.

So, I blurted out-How is everyone's HIV. Everyone at the table had a different response. The guy sitting to the left, looked at me big eyed and mouth wide open, as if I'd said something wrong. The guy sitting to my right, screamed out my name-"BRADLEY! Why would you bring that up like that?" His face expressed his disgust with the subject. He quickly rose from the chair and stormed out of the living room. The guy sitting across from me, replied, "Now that is something to clear a room."

Oddly, the first guy to leave the table, has held a grudge against me since that day. We still haven't spoken since last summer. It's Summer again. I didn't even get a chance to attend his mother's funeral because of his discomfort with a conversation about HIV, at a table with other people who each are living with the virus.

As an HIV/AIDS Educator and Counselor, which I held such a position for Detroit Community Health Connection, Inc. in 2000. I found the job stressful. After all, who was I to take the initiative to play government advocate to try and encourage grown men and women to make health changes in their daily lives. I also felt uncomfortable listening to so many different sob stories about families turning their backs on family because the gay man or lesbian female, was victimized by some stranger who was coward and refused to be an adult to help protect others from being victimized.

Like many of you reading this book; you, too, may feel threatened and unloved by family and friends who reject you because of your life style or sexual orientation. Please don't allow others ignorance to impede upon your joy and happiness.

It's one thing to be gay, lesbian, or bi-sexual, and be neglected or discriminated against by strangers. But when family discriminate against you, it's a different story.

Luckily, there are groups in major cities that offer daily and weekly sessions to connect with others who may be helpful in providing the resources and encouragement, you need to set yourself free from the ignorance, you may be forced to live around. Take a brief moment and log online to research HIV groups in your area. If you don't discover any, search for the nearest HIV/AIDS resource agency who can provide the guidance, you seek. If all else fails, please feel free to connect with me. You can do so by emailing me at positivelightforliving@gmail.com. Be sure to put: POZ, in the subject.

Remembering to Be Honest

Now that you've tested positive there's no longer a need to be afraid of telling the truth. Take it from me; sharing your HIV diagnosis with sexual partners and strangers, you meet at the bar gets much easier as time passes on. Just to prove it, I want to share why I found it so compelling to evoke others to feel comfortable about telling the truth.

Ironically, one night while having a nice time at a local night club, I met this very distinguishing looking fellow who was extremely attractive. As a result, I approached him and asked, if he wanted a drink. Of course, he accepted the kind offer.

Afterwards, while talking and getting to know one another; I noticed, he had a sore on his lip. Grant it, at first, I thought it was merely a cold sore, something that was curable. However, when I asked him what it was, he informed me it was herpes. Shocked, I was instantly taken aback.

53

Moreover, I was surprised at how honest he was.

As a result, I informed him that I was HIV positive. Funny, you should've seen the look on his face. It was as if he'd won the lottery. So, I asked him why the expression of surprise. His response, "I'm HIV positive, too."

After sharing a few spins out on the dance floor, we eventually decided to go back to his place. Not to have sex. But to finish discussing how fearful we both had previously been about sharing our diagnosis with others.

After a few dates, he and I took it to another level. In fact, doing so gave us both a life time of passionate memories. But the best part about it was that, we'd already cleared the air, which allowed us the gift of letting our guard down and enjoying one another's company completely; without feeling guilty after doing so.

Therefore, whenever you feel as though you're the only one living with this virus; think again. The very person you may find yourself attracted to and afraid to share your HIV diagnosis with, might perhaps also be infected and afraid to share their diagnosis with you.

An Exclusive Interview with Bradley Fowler, MA, MSc.

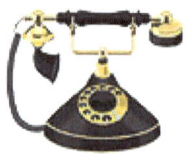

Q. So, Bradley, please tell me how long you've been HIV positive?

A. For over ten years.

Q. Are you on any medication to help suppress the virus?

A. Yes, I'm on one pill a day-Genvoya. I also take Marinol and smoke one marijuana cigarette daily.

Q. Since testing positive, how high has your viral load gotten?

A. My viral load has never exceeded 7,000 copies.

Q. What was the highest CD4 count you've had?

A. 1200.

Q. Are you still conducting HIV counseling in your community?

A. Not clinically. Actually, I've stepped out of the traditional office and found solace working from home online. Doing so allots me the opportunity to focus more on completing my Doctor of Education in Education Administration. I also find connecting with individuals online less stressful and impersonal.

Q. Are you involved with anyone presently?

A. Yes.

Q. Was it hard to find someone to embrace you after testing positive?

A. No. In fact, the man, I'm dating now is the same man I've been dating for 21 years. We agreed to get tested together. Unfortunately, I tested positive; he didn't.

Q. How does being HIV positive weigh on your sex life?

A. Honestly, it hasn't hindered it much. My partner is a bottom. So, I refrain from exchanging bodily fluids.

Q. Do you wear condoms during sex?

A. Occasionally; I'm not a fan of condoms.

Q. How does being HIV positive affect your life?

A. Over the years, I've learned to take it one-day-at-a-time. And honestly, it's no different than if I had some other ailment. Although I've been getting headaches a lot lately. I recently discovered it was my medicine causing them. In addition, I've learned to force myself to fight the mental set backs of being positive. Often, depression attacks those living with HIV. So instead, I've learned to throw myself into various hobbies. Plus, I pamper my cats. Even more interesting, when I'm feeling a little down I've learned to force myself to focus on positive thinking and self-talk, which enables me to move forth in whatever I seek to do. After all, that is the only way I have ever dealt with this virus. That's why today, I pretty much have a "just do it" attitude.

Q. You seem to have a strong grip on being HIV positive; have you ever experienced any set-backs?

A. The only set back I've really had, is not being able to enjoy my social life, as I once did. Nowadays, I'm so busy building a foundation around my Doctor of Education degree studies and trying to develop a new platform for religious studies (e.g. https://www.thegren.com), which is stressful. However, I've learned that it's best to focus on what's most entertaining for me; and in doing so, I'm able to create a better dialogue for my readers.

Q. And does your companion convey much support about you being HIV positive?

A. Yes, we're very close knit and private; we don't have a social network of friends. But again, this is why I enjoy writing. It tends to give me a chance to entertain others who, too, are HIV positive and seeking positive mediums to empower themselves. Plus, sharing my knowledge has allotted me the opportunity to help countless others overcome their fear and discomfort about disclosure. In addition, my partner is the force behind helping me finish my Doctor of Education.

Q. Have you written any other types of books?

A. Yes.

Q. I understand, you gained your HIV educator and counseling certification with the State of Michigan Department of Community Health, what was that like?

A. It was a three-day course that involved communication skills, time consuming studying, testing, and evaluations. In fact, I'm scheduled to update my certification in the coming weeks, online via the Michigan Department of Community Health Web site.

Q. Before I close is there anything else you would like to share with your readers?

A. Yes, please feel free to contact me with questions, concerns, and flirts at: positivelightforliving@gmail.com Be sure to put: POZ in the subject box.

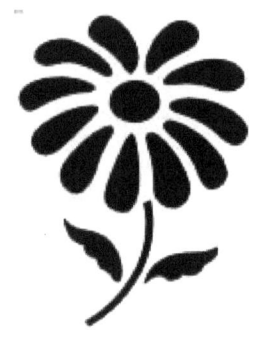

References

CDC.gov. (2019). Statistics. Website: https://www.cdc.gov/hiv/statistics/overview/ataglance.html

UNAIDS.org. (2019). Global Statistics. Website: https://www.hiv.gov/hiv-basics/overview/data-and-trends/global-statistics

The Guardian.com. (2019). HIV Carriers Face Microchip Implants in Indonesia's Papua Province. Website: https://www.theguardian.com/world/2008/Nov/24/indonesia-aids

POZ.com (2019). POZ Personals. Website: https://www.poz.com

www.ingramcontent.com/pod-product-compliance
Lightning Source LLC
Chambersburg PA
CBHW050816290526
45792CB00001B/142